Bipul Nath
LilaKanta Nath
Bhaskar Mazumder

Gastric Floating Microcapsules of Metformin HCl

Bipul Nath
LilaKanta Nath
Bhaskar Mazumder

# Gastric Floating Microcapsules of Metformin HCl

Methods, Evaluation and Applications

LAP LAMBERT Academic Publishing

**Impressum/Imprint (nur für Deutschland/only for Germany)**
Bibliografische Information der Deutschen Nationalbibliothek: Die Deutsche Nationalbibliothek verzeichnet diese Publikation in der Deutschen Nationalbibliografie; detaillierte bibliografische Daten sind im Internet über http://dnb.d-nb.de abrufbar.
Alle in diesem Buch genannten Marken und Produktnamen unterliegen warenzeichen-, marken- oder patentrechtlichem Schutz bzw. sind Warenzeichen oder eingetragene Warenzeichen der jeweiligen Inhaber. Die Wiedergabe von Marken, Produktnamen, Gebrauchsnamen, Handelsnamen, Warenbezeichnungen u.s.w. in diesem Werk berechtigt auch ohne besondere Kennzeichnung nicht zu der Annahme, dass solche Namen im Sinne der Warenzeichen- und Markenschutzgesetzgebung als frei zu betrachten wären und daher von jedermann benutzt werden dürften.

Coverbild: www.ingimage.com

Verlag: LAP LAMBERT Academic Publishing GmbH & Co. KG
Dudweiler Landstr. 99, 66123 Saarbrücken, Deutschland
Telefon +49 681 3720-310, Telefax +49 681 3720-3109
Email: info@lap-publishing.com

Approved by: Dibrugarh, Dibrugarh University, Diss. 2007

Herstellung in Deutschland:
Schaltungsdienst Lange o.H.G., Berlin
Books on Demand GmbH, Norderstedt
Reha GmbH, Saarbrücken
Amazon Distribution GmbH, Leipzig
**ISBN: 978-3-8454-7680-3**

**Imprint (only for USA, GB)**
Bibliographic information published by the Deutsche Nationalbibliothek: The Deutsche Nationalbibliothek lists this publication in the Deutsche Nationalbibliografie; detailed bibliographic data are available in the Internet at http://dnb.d-nb.de.
Any brand names and product names mentioned in this book are subject to trademark, brand or patent protection and are trademarks or registered trademarks of their respective holders. The use of brand names, product names, common names, trade names, product descriptions etc. even without a particular marking in this works is in no way to be construed to mean that such names may be regarded as unrestricted in respect of trademark and brand protection legislation and could thus be used by anyone.

Cover image: www.ingimage.com

Publisher: LAP LAMBERT Academic Publishing GmbH & Co. KG
Dudweiler Landstr. 99, 66123 Saarbrücken, Germany
Phone +49 681 3720-310, Fax +49 681 3720-3109
Email: info@lap-publishing.com

Printed in the U.S.A.
Printed in the U.K. by (see last page)
**ISBN: 978-3-8454-7680-3**

Copyright © 2011 by the author and LAP LAMBERT Academic Publishing GmbH & Co. KG and licensors
All rights reserved. Saarbrücken 2011

**Preface**

This book represents a unique attempt to overview the full range of approaches to discovering, selecting, and designing a dosage form for gastric retention of therapeutic moieties that have site specific absorption limitation problems. This volume is unique in that it seeks to cover possible approaches to the pharmaceutical techniques as broadly as possible while not just doing so in a superficial manner. I hope that this edition of the book would satisfy and useful to all those working in or entering the field of pharmacy. The pharmaceutical industry has seen several waves of consolidation with each successive year. The economic pressures on the industry have been increasing due to political policies and dwindling supply of new chemical entities. The surge in expiration of patents has given opportunities to the generic drug industry as never seen before and the trend will continue for some time to come. To maintain market share and remain in the forefront of technological advances, a number of different dosage forms utilizing different technologies have been explored. In today world, the Pharmaceutical Industry is caught in between downward pressure on prices and increase cost of a successful drug discovery and development due to strict and stringent regulations. This has prompted a more research on fabrication of the existing drug molecules to improve its performance on safety, efficacy and patient compliance. Prolonged gastric retention improves bioavailability, reduces drug waste, and improves solubility for drugs that are less soluble in a high pH environment. It has applications also for local drug delivery to the stomach and proximal small intestines.

This book is written with special focus on the principal mechanism of floatation and the approaches to achieve gastric retention. The author has also highlighted the formulation of floating microcapsules of metformin HCl by slight modification of emulsion solvent evaporation method with a view to increase its bioavailability. Although, extended release, sustained release metformin tablet formulations are in the market, it cannot improve the bioavailability of metformin HCl. As these formulations disintegrate quickly and releases the drug very fast and the desired controlled effect cannot be achieved and thus cause great fluctuations in plasma drug levels. But, controlled release floating microcapsules of metformin HCl made of cellulose acetate butyrate and eudragit RL100 polymer using emulsion solvent evaporation method have sufficient buoyancy to float over gastric contents and thus improve the bioavailability of the drug.

The author hope the knowledge provided through this book will be invaluable for selecting the appropriate technology, while keeping in mind regulatory requirements and cost effectiveness of dosage forms.

## *Acknowledgement*

I would like to acknowledge the support and cooperation of few of my teachers contributing throughout the completion of this book; and to them I offer a most sincere thank you. Without their suggestion and timely guidance, this book would not have gone to print. I would like to give special mention to Mr. Manzir Sarma Kotoki, Asst. Professor, Department of Pharmaceutical Sciences, Himachal, Baddi (India), Assam for his invaluable support, encouragement, and constant supervision in successful completion during this project. I wish to express my sincere thanks to Dr. Dipak Chetia, Head, Department of Pharmaceutical Sciences, Dibrugarh Unieversity for providing departmental facilities and his kind co-operations and suggestions. I also express my profound gratefulness to all my beloved teachers, Department of Pharmaceutical Sciences, Dibrugarh University for their sincere teaching's, co-operation and help in every aspect of my work. Finally, I owe my loving acknowledgement to my parents and wife Anusmita Dutta for their love, encouragement and invaluable support throughout the completion of my work.

A special recognition goes to the Ms. Tatiana Melnic, Acquisition Editor, LAP Lambert Academic Publishing GmbH & Co. KG Dudweiler Landstr. 99, 66123 Saarbrucken, Germany. It was with his encouragement that i was driven to write this book.

# Table of Contents

| | |
|---|---|
| Preface | 1 |
| Acknowledgement | 2 |
| 1.1 Introduction | 5-6 |
| 1.2 Basic Gastrointestinal Tract Physiology | 6 |
|     1.2.1 Factors to be considered in the design of Gastro-retentive Drug Delivery System | 6-8 |
| 1.3 Fundamentals of Gastro retentive Drug Delivery System | 8-10 |
| 1.4 Suitable Drug Candidates for Gastro retentive Drug Delivery System | 10-12 |
| 1.5 Approaches to Design Floating Dosage Forms | 12 |
|     1.5.1 Single-Unit Dosage Forms | 13-14 |
|     1.5.2 Multiple-Unit Dosage Forms | 14-15 |
| 1.6 Classification of Floating Drug Delivery Systems (FDDS) | 15 |
|     1.6.1 Effervescent Floating Dosage Forms | 15-19 |
|     1.6.2 Non-Effervescent Floating Dosage Forms | 19-23 |
| 2.1 Fundamental considerations for microencapsulation of therapeutic agents | 23 |
|     2.1.1 Core material | 23 |
|     2.1.2 Coating material | 23-24 |
|     2.1.3 Methods for preparation of perforated floating microcapsules | 24-25 |
| 3.1 Evaluation of the floating microcapsules | 25 |
|     3.1.1 Yield of microcapsules | 25 |
|     3.1.2 Particle size analysis | 26 |
|     3.1.3 Viscosity of the polymer solutions | 26-27 |
|     3.1.4 Density determinations | 27 |
|     3.1.5 Bulk density | 27 |
|     3.1.6 Angle of contact | 27 |
|     3.1.7 Drug entrapment efficiency | 27-28 |
|     3.1.8 In vitro Evaluation of Floating Ability | 28-29 |
|     3.1.9 Scanning Electron Microscopy (SEM) | 29-30 |
|     3.1.10 Fourier Transform Infrared Spectroscopy (FT-IR) | 30-32 |
|     3.1.11 Differential Scanning Calorimetry (DSC) | 32 |
|     3.1.12 X-ray powder Diffractometry | 32-33 |
|     3.1.13 Dissolution characteristics of Metformin HCl floating microcapsules | 33-37 |
|     3.1.14 Release Kinetics | 37 |
| 4.1 Conclusions | 39 |
| References | 39-45 |

**Dedicated**

**To**

**My parents**

**Shri Sukladhar Nath and**

**Smt. Putuli Nath**

## 1.1 Introduction

Despite tremendous advancement in the drug delivery system, oral route remains the preferred route for the administration of therapeutic agents and because of low cost therapy and ease of administration leads to higher levels of patient compliance. But, several difficulties are faced in designing oral controlled release systems for better absorption and enhanced bioavailability. Conventional oral dosage forms such as tablets, capsules, provide specific drug concentration in systemic circulation without offering any control over drug delivery and also cause great fluctuations in plasma drug levels. The design of oral controlled drug delivery system should be primarily aimed to achieve more predictable and increased bioavailability. Approx. 50% of the drug delivery system available in the market is oral DDS and these systems have more advantage due to patient acceptance and ease of administration.

This ideal system should have single oral dose for the whole duration of treatment and it should deliver the drug directly at the specific site. Controlled release implies the predictability and reproducibility to control the drug release and drug concentration in the target tissue and optimization of the therapeutic effect of a drug by controlling its release in the body with lower and less frequent dose. A well designed controlled drug delivery system can overcome some of the problems of conventional therapy and enhance the therapeutic efficacy of a given drug. To obtain maximum therapeutic efficacy, it becomes necessary to deliver the agent to the target tissue in the optimal amount in the right period of time there by causing little toxicity and minimal side effects [1].

Although the single unit floating dosage form have been extensively studied, these single unit dosage form have the disadvantage of a release all or nothing emptying process while the multiple unit particulate system pass through the GIT to avoid the vagaries of gastric emptying and thus release the drug more uniformly [2]. The uniform distribution of these multiple unit dosage forms along the GIT could result in more reproducible drug absorption and reduced risk of local irritation; this gave birth to oral controlled drug delivery and led to development of gastro retentive floating micro spheres/microcapsules [3, 4]. Several difficulties are faced in designing oral controlled release systems for better absorption and enhanced bioavailability. One of such difficulties is the inability to confine the dosage form in the desired area of the gastrointestinal tract. But, floating micro spheres/microcapsules can deliver a therapeutic substance to the target site in a sustained controlled release fashion. Gastro retentive systems can remain in the gastric region for several hours and hence significantly prolong the gastric residence time of drugs. Prolonged gastric retention improves bioavailability, reduces drug waste, and improves solubility for drugs that are less soluble in a high pH environment. It has applications also for local drug delivery to the stomach and proximal small intestines. Gastro retention helps to provide better availability of new products with new therapeutic possibilities and substantial benefits for patients [5, 6].

## 1.2 Basic Gastrointestinal Tract Physiology

To comprehend the considerations taken in the design of GRDFs and to evaluate their performance the relevant anatomy and physiology of the gastrointestinal tract must be fully understood. The stomach is situated in the left upper part of the abdominal cavity immediately under the diaphragm [7]. Its size varies according to the amount of distention: up to 1500 ml [8] following a meal; after food has emptied, a 'collapsed' state is obtained with a resting volume of only 25–50 ml [9]. The stomach is composed of the following parts: fundus, above the opening of the esophagus into the stomach; body, the central part; and antrum. The pylorus is an anatomical sphincter situated between the most terminal antrum and the duodenum. The fundus and the body store food temporarily, secrete digestive juices and propulse chyme, a milky mixture of food with gastric juices, to the antrum. The antrum grinds and triturates food particles and regulates the secretion of hydrochloric acid as well as the emptying of food [9].

Fasting gastric pH is usually steady and approximates 2, but there are short periods of 766 min characterized by higher values. Food buffers and neutralizes gastric acid, thus increasing the pH up to about 6.5. After meal-ingestion is completed, the pH rapidly falls back below 5 and then gradually declines to fasting state values over a period of a few hours [10]. In the elderly population approximately 20% are hypochlorhydric i.e. with reduced but not absent gastric secretion, whereas the remainders have acid production similar to young people [11]. The pyloric sphincter has a diameter of 12.867 mm in humans [6, 7] and acts as a sieve as well as a mechanical stricture to the passage of large particles [9]. The duodenal pH is 6.1 [10] and its epithelial surface contains transporters for peptides and metals [12]. The transit time in the duodenum is relatively short, less than 1 min [3]. The small intestine has a large surface area, which is comparable to the area of a basketball court, 463 m$^2$. This is the main reason it is the primary absorption site of water, ions, vitamins and nutrients such as amino acids, fats and sugars. In addition, the digestion of fats, peptides and sugars occurs in this segment of the gastrointestinal tract [7]. The pH of the small intestine is 6–7 [8]. The transit time in the small intestine of 3±1 h [13], is relatively constant and is unaffected by food [8].

## 1.2.1 Factors to be considered in the design of Gastro retentive Drug Delivery System

Gastric residence time of an oral dosage form is affected by several factors. To pass through the pyloric valve into the small intestine the particle size should be in the range of 1 to 2 mm and the pH of the stomach in fasting state is ~1.5 to 2.0 and in fed state is 2.0 to 6.0. A large volume of water administered with an oral dosage form raises the pH of stomach contents to 6.0 to 9.0. Stomach doesn't get time to produce sufficient acid when the liquid empties the stomach; hence generally basic drugs have a better chance of dissolving in fed state than in a fasting state.

The rate of gastric emptying depends mainly on viscosity, volume, and caloric content of meals. Nutritive density of meals helps determine gastric emptying time. It does not make any difference whether the meal has high protein, fat, or carbohydrate content as long as the caloric content is the same. However, increase in acidity and caloric value slows down gastric emptying time. Biological factors such as age, body mass index (BMI), gender, posture, and diseased states (diabetes, Chron's disease) influence gastric emptying. In the case of elderly persons, gastric emptying is slowed down. Generally females have slower gastric emptying rates than males. Stress increases gastric emptying rates while depression slows it down [2]

Gastric Volume is important for dissolution of dosage form in vivo. The resting volume of the stomach is 25 to 50 mL. Volume of liquids administered affects the gastric emptying time. When volume is large, the emptying is faster. Fluids taken at body temperature leave the stomach faster than colder or warmer fluids. Studies have revealed that gastric emptying of a dosage form in the fed state can also be influenced by its size. Small-size tablets leave the stomach during the digestive phase while the large-size tablets are emptied during the housekeeping waves.

Timmermans and Andre [14] studied the effect of size of floating and nonfloating dosage forms on gastric emptying and concluded that the floating units remained buoyant on gastric fluids. These are less likely to be expelled from the stomach compared with the nonfloating units, which lie in the antrum region and are propelled by the peristaltic waves.

Several formulation parameters can affect the gastric residence time. More reliable gastric emptying patterns are observed for multiparticulate formulations as compared with single unit formulations, which suffer from "all or none concept." As the units of multiparticulate systems are distributed freely throughout the gastrointestinal tract, their transport is affected to a lesser extent by the transit time of food compared with single unit formulation [17].

Size and shape of dosage unit also affect the gastric emptying. Garg and Sharma [18] reported that tetrahedron and ring-shaped devices have a better gastric residence time as compared with other shapes. The diameter of the dosage unit is also equally important as a formulation parameter. Dosage forms having a diameter of more than 7.5 mm show a better gastric residence time compared with one having 9.9 mm.

The density of a dosage form also affects the gastric emptying rate. A buoyant dosage form having a density of less than that of the gastric fluids floats. Since it is away from the pyloric sphincter, the dosage unit is retained in the stomach for a prolonged period.

Javed et al [19] studied the effect of buoyancy, posture, and nature of meals on the gastric emptying process in vivo using gamma scintigraphy. To perform these studies, floating and nonfloating capsules of 3 different sizes having a diameter of 4.8 mm (small units), 7.5 mm (medium units), and 9.9 mm (large units), were formulated. On comparison of floating and nonfloating dosage units, it was concluded that regardless of their sizes the floating dosage units remained buoyant on the gastric contents throughout their residence in the gastrointestinal tract, while the nonfloating dosage units sank and remained in the lower part of the stomach. Floating units away from the gastroduodenal junction were protected from the peristaltic waves during digestive phase while the nonfloating forms stayed close to the pylorus and were subjected to propelling and retropelling waves of the digestive phase (Figure 1). It was also observed that of the floating and nonfloating units, the floating units were had a longer gastric residence time for small and medium units while no significant difference was seen between the 2 types of large unit dosage forms. Gamma Scintigraphic studies revealed that the optimized HBS capsule was retained in the gastric region (stomach) for a prolonged period and the study of pharmacokinetic studies showed an increase in AUC as compared to immediate release capsules of metformin.

## 1.2 Fundamentals of Gastro retentive Drug Delivery System

Over the last three decades, various attempts have been made to retain the dosage form in the stomach as away of increasing retention time.
- High-density system having density of 3 g/cm3, are retained in the rugae of the stomach. The major disadvantage with such system is that it is technically difficult to manufacture them with a large amount of drug (>50%) and to achieve the required density of 2.4-2.8 g/cm3.

- Swelling systems are capable of swelling to assize that prevents their passage through the pylorus; as a result the dosage form is remained in the stomach for longer period of time. Upon coming in contact with gastric fluid, the polymer imbibes water and swells.
- Bio/muco-adhesive systems bind to the gastric epithelial cell surface or mucin and extend the GRT by increasing the intimacy and duration of contact between the dosage form and the biological membrane.
- Floating/low density systems are low density systems that have sufficient buoyancy to float over gastric contents, and the drug is released slowly at the desired rate, which results increased gastro-retention time and reduces fluctuations in plasma drug concentration.

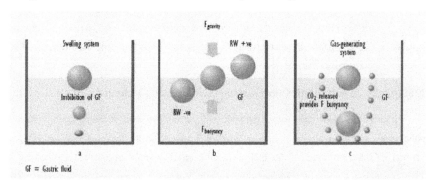

**Figure 1.2 Various forms of oral floating drug delivery system.**

Such GFDDS are important for drugs that are degraded in the intestine or for drugs like antacid or certain antibiotics, enzymes that act locally in the stomach. If the drugs are poorly soluble in the intestine due to alkaline pH and then it's retention in the gastric region may increase the solubility before they are emptied, resulting in increased bioavailability.

Gastric emptying of dosage forms is an extremely variable process and ability to prolong and control the emptying time is a valuable asset for dosage forms, which reside in the stomach for a longer period of time than conventional dosage forms. Several difficulties are faced in designing controlled release systems for better absorption and enhanced bioavailability. It is widely acknowledged that the extent of gastrointestinal tract drug absorption is related to contact time with the small intestinal mucosa. Thus, small intestinal transit time is an important parameter for drugs that are incompletely absorbed.

Gastro retentive systems can remain in the gastric region for several hours and hence significantly prolong the gastric residence time of drugs. Prolonged gastric retention improves bioavailability, reduces drug waste, and improves solubility for drugs that are less soluble in a high pH environment. It has applications also for local drug delivery to the stomach and proximal small intestines. Gastro retention helps to provide better availability of new products with new therapeutic possibilities and substantial benefits for patients.

The controlled gastric retention of solid dosage forms may be achieved by the mechanisms of mucoadhesion [20], flotation [21, 22], sedimentation, [23] expansion [24, 25], modified shape systems [26, 27] or by the simultaneous administration of pharmacological agents that delay gastric emptying. Based on these approaches, classification of floating drug delivery systems (FDDS) has been described in detail. In vivo/in scientists to assess the efficiency and application of such systems have discussed vitro evaluation of FDDS. Several recent examples have been reported showing the efficiency of such systems for drugs with bioavailability problems.

## 1.4 Suitable Drug Candidates for Gastro retentive Drug Delivery System

Various drugs have their greatest therapeutic effect when released in the stomach, particularly when the release is prolonged in a continuous, controlled manner. Drugs delivered in this manner have a lower level of side effects and provide their therapeutic effects without the need for repeated dosages or with a low dosage frequency. Sustained release in the stomach is also useful for therapeutic agents that the stomach does not readily absorb, since sustained release prolongs the contact time of the agent in the stomach or in the upper part of the small intestine, which is where absorption occurs and contact time is limited. Under normal or average conditions, for example, material passes through the small intestine in as little as 1-3 hours. In general, appropriate candidates for CRGRDF are molecules that have poor colonic absorption but are characterized by better absorption properties at the upper parts of the GIT:

1. Narrow absorption window in GI tract, e.g., riboflavin and levodopa
2. Primarily absorbed from stomach and upper part of GIT, e.g., calcium supplements, chlordiazepoxide and cinnarizine.
3. Drugs that act locally in the stomach, e.g., antacids, ranitidine, cimetidine and misoprostol.
4. Drugs that degrade in the colon, e.g., ranitidine HCl and metronidazole.
5. Drugs that disturb normal colonic bacteria, e.g., amoxicillin trihydrate.

Other drugs that act locally in the stomach are lansoprazole, omeprazole, rabeprazole etc.

Lansoprazole is a powerful inhibitor of gastric acid, and can totally abolish HCl secretion both in resting as well as in stimulated conditions. They are inactive at neutral ph but at ph<5 rearranges to two cationic form that react co-valently with –SH group of H+K+ATPase. So, it require selective local delivery of the drug to the stomach, where gastroretentive dosage form will retain the drug in the stomach for longer period of time [28].

Cimetidine when administered orally adequately absorbed and the bioavailability is 60-80% due to its first-pass hepatic metabolism. It has short serum half-life and about 30% of the administered dose is slowly inactivated by the livers microsomal mixed function oxygenase system. Srivastava et al [29] reported Cimetidine loaded floating micro spheres of HPMC and ethyl cellulose. The prepared micro spheres exhibited prolonged drug release (up to 8hrs) and remain buoyant for 8-9 hrs, which in turn overcome the bioavailability problem of the drug.

Various antibiotics are better absorbed in empty stomach such as Tetracycline, doxycycline, amoxicillin etc. Clarithromycin is a class of macrolide antibiotic, which is more active against gram positive legionella, mycoplasma, pneumonia, H.pylori infections are better absorbed in acidic conditions. The site specific delivery of drugs for the treatment of infectious diseases such as ameobiasis (metronidazole), Helicobacter pylori ( and it would be very much useful in reducing the relapse of these diseases and for minimizing the side effects associated with the systemic absorption of these drugs.[30,31]

Another drug which is promising for gastroretentive drug delivery system is metformin HCl. Metformin, is an oral antidiabetic drug in the biguanide class. It is the first-line drug of choice for the treatment of type 2 diabetes, in particular, in overweight and obese people and those with normal kidney function. Evidence is also mounting for its efficacy in gestational diabetes, although safety concerns still preclude its widespread use in this setting. It is also used in the treatment of polycystic ovary syndrome, and has been investigated for other diseases where insulin resistance may be an important factor.

When prescribed appropriately, metformin causes few adverse effects the most common is gastrointestinal upset and is associated with a low risk of hypoglycemia. Lactic acidosis (a buildup of lactate in the blood) can be a serious concern in overdose and when it is prescribed to people with contraindications, but otherwise, there is no significant risk. Metformin helps reduce LDL cholesterol and triglyceride levels, and is not associated with weight gain, and is the only antidiabetic drug that has been conclusively shown to prevent the cardiovascular complications of diabetes. As of 2010, metformin is one of only two oral antidiabetics in the World Health Organization Model List of Essential Medicines (the other being glibenclamide) [32]. First synthesized and found to reduce blood sugar in the 1920s, metformin was forgotten for the next two decades as research shifted to insulin and other antidiabetic drugs. Interest in metformin was rekindled in the late 1940s after several reports that it could reduce blood sugar levels in people, and in 1957, French physician Jean Sterne published the first clinical trial of metformin as a treatment for diabetes. It was introduced to the United Kingdom in 1958, Canada in 1972, and the United States in 1995. Metformin is now believed to be the most widely prescribed antidiabetic drug in the world; in the United States alone, more than 48 million prescriptions were filled in 2010 for its generic formulations. [33, 34]

Stepensky et al [35] concluded that absolute oral bioavailability of metformin HCl is 50-60% due to its site-specific absorption limitations. It is safe drug and it has a half-life of 1.5-3 hrs. It is not absorbed completely and gives low bioavailability problem. Almost 80-100% of the drug is excreted unchanged. The total daily requirement of metformin HCl is 1.5-3g/day. Henceforth, there being high incidence of GI side effects and toxicity. Therefore, there are continued efforts to improve the pharmaceutical formulation of metformin hydrochloride in order to achieve an optimal therapy. These efforts mainly focus on controlled/slow release of the drug including the sophisticated gastro- retentive systems. However, bioavailability of the drug has been found to be reduced further with controlled release dosage forms, probably due to the fact that passage of the controlled release single unit dosage forms from absorption region of the drug is faster than its release and most of the drug released at the colon where metformin hydrochloride is poorly absorbed [35].

Controlled release formulation suitable for metformin hydrochloride, therefore, should be a gastro-retentive dosage form, which releases the drug slowly in the stomach for gradual absorption in the intestines. The slow but complete drug release in the stomach is expected to increase bioavailability of the drug as well its complete utilization which may results to, lower dose and GI side effects. Multi unit dosage forms are considered to release the drug at a controlled rate and remain in the stomach for a prolonged period with much less chance of dose dumping. Furthermore they are supposed to cause less gastric adverse reactions and are insensitive to concomitant food intake, thereby reducing inter and intra-patient variability and increasing the predictability of the dosage form.

## 1.4 Approaches to Design Floating Dosage Forms

The following approaches have been used for the design of floating dosage forms of single- and multiple-unit systems [40]

### 1.5.1 Single-Unit Dosage Forms

In Low-density approach [22] the globular shells apparently having lower density than that of gastric fluid can be used as a carrier for drug for its controlled release. A buoyant dosage form can also be obtained by using a fluid-filled system that floats in the stomach. In coated shells [37] popcorn, pop rice, and polystyrol have been exploited as drug carriers. Sugar polymeric materials such as met acrylic polymer and cellulose acetate phthalate have been used to undercoat these shells. These are further coated with a drug-polymer mixture. The polymer of choice can be either ethyl cellulose or hydroxypropyl cellulose depending on the type of release desired. Finally, the product floats on the gastric fluid while releasing the drug gradually over a prolonged duration.

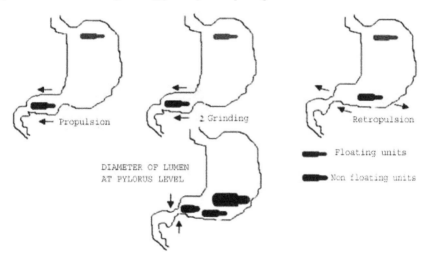

**Figure 1.4 Intragastric residence positions of floating and nonfloating units.**

Fluid filled floating chamber [38] type of dosage forms includes incorporation of a gas-filled floatation chamber into a microporous component that houses a drug reservoir. Apertures or openings are present along the top and bottom walls through which the gastrointestinal tract fluid enters to dissolve the drug. The other two walls in contact with the fluid are sealed so that the undissolved drug remains therein. The fluid present could be air, under partial vacuum or any other suitable gas, liquid, or solid having an appropriate specific gravity and an inert behavior. The device is of swallowable size, remains afloat within the stomach for a prolonged time, and after the complete release the shell disintegrates, passes off to the intestine, and is eliminated. Hydrodynamically balanced systems (HBS) are designed to prolong the stay of the dosage form in the gastro intestinal tract and aid in enhancing the absorption. Such systems are best suited for drugs having a better solubility in acidic environment and also for the drugs having specific site of absorption in the upper part of the small intestine. To remain in the stomach for a prolonged period of time the dosage form must have a bulk density of less than 1. It should stay in the stomach, maintain its structural integrity, and release drug constantly from the dosage form. The success of HBS capsule as a better system is best exemplified with chlordiazeopoxide hydrochloride. The drug is a classical example of a solubility problem wherein it exhibits a 4000-fold difference in solubility going from pH 3 to 6 (the solubility of chlordiazepoxide hydrochloride is 150 mg/mL and is ~0.1 mg/mL at neutral pH).

Javed Ali et al [39] develop a hydrodynamically balanced system of metformin as a single unit floating capsule. Various grades of low-density polymers were used for the formulation of this system. It was concluded on the basis of buoyancy and in vitro release kinetics that optimized formulation containing 500 mg of metformin granulated with 5% of ethyl cellulose, and 150 mg of HPMC K4M (extragranular) gave the best in vitro release of 97% in 12 h in simulated gastric fluid at pH 3. The release of metformin from the matrix formulation followed zero order release kinetics. Gamma Scintigraphic studies revealed that the optimized HBS capsule was retained in the gastric region (stomach) for a prolonged period and the study of pharmacokinetic studies showed an increase in AUC as compared to immediate release capsules of metformin.

Various types of tablets (bilayered and matrix) have been shown to have floatable characteristics. Some of the polymers used are hydroxypropyl cellulose, hydroxypropyl methylcellulose, crosspovidone, sodium carboxymethyl cellulose, and ethyl cellulose. Self-correcting floatable asymmetric configuration drug delivery system [40] employs a disproportionate 3-layer matrix technology to control drug release.

The 3-layer principle has been improved by development of an asymmetric configuration drug delivery system in order to modulate the release extent and achieve zero-order release kinetics by initially maintaining a constant area at the diffusing front with subsequent dissolution/erosion toward the completion of the release process. The system was designed in such a manner that it floated to prolong gastric residence time in vivo, resulting in longer total transit time within the gastrointestinal tract environment with maximum absorptive capacity and consequently greater bioavailability. This particular characteristic would be applicable to drugs that have pH dependent solubility, a narrow window of absorption, and are absorbed by active transport from either the proximal or distal portion of the small intestine. Single-unit formulations are associated with problems such as sticking together or being obstructed in the gastrointestinal tract, which may have a potential danger of producing irritation.

### 1.5.2 Multiple-Unit Dosage Forms

The purpose of designing multiple-unit dosage form is to develop a reliable formulation that has all the advantages of a single-unit form and also is devoid of any of the above mentioned disadvantages of single-unit formulations. In pursuit of this endeavor many multiple-unit floatable dosage forms have been designed. Microspheres have high loading capacity and many polymers have been used such as albumin, gelatin, starch, polymethacrylate, polyacrylamine, and polyalkylcyanoacrylate. Spherical polymeric microsponges also referred to as "micro balloons," have been prepared. Microspheres have a characteristic internal hollow structure and show an excellent in vitro floatability [41]. In Carbon dioxide–generating multiple-unit oral formulations [42] several devices with features that extend, unfold, or are inflated by carbon dioxide generated in the devices after administration have been described in the recent patent literature. These dosage forms are excluded from the passage of the pyloric sphincter if a diameter of ~12 to 18 mm in their expanded state is exceeded.

## 1.6 Classification of Floating Drug Delivery Systems (FDDS)

Floating drug delivery systems are classified depending on the mechanism of buoyancy: effervescent and non-effervescent systems.

### 1.6.1 Effervescent Floating Dosage Forms

These are matrix types of systems prepared with the help of swell able polymers such as methylcellulose and chitosan and various effervescent compounds, e.g., sodium bicarbonate, tartaric acid, and citric acid. They are formulated in such a way that when in contact with the acidic gastric contents, $CO_2$ is liberated and get entrapped in swollen hydrocolloids, which provides buoyancy to the dosage forms (Figure 1.6, A and B).

Ichikawa et al [42] developed a new multiple type of floating dosage system composed of effervescent layers and swellable membrane layers coated on sustained release pills. The inner layer of effervescent agents containing sodium bicarbonate and tartaric acid was divided into 2 sublayers to avoid direct contact between the 2 agents. These sublayers were surrounded by a swellable polymer membrane containing polyvinyl acetate and purified shellac. When this system was immersed in the buffer at 37°C, it settled down and the solution permeated into the effervescent layer through the outer swellable membrane. $CO_2$ was generated by the neutralization reaction between the 2 effervescent agents, producing swollen pills (like balloons) with a density less than 1.0 g/mL. It was found that the system had good floating ability independent of pH and viscosity and the drug (para-amino benzoic acid) released in a sustained manner [42] (Figure 1.6, A and B).

Ichikawa et al [43] developed floating capsules composed of a plurality of granules that have different residence times in the stomach and consist of an inner foamable layer of gasgenerating agents. This layer was further divided into 2 sublayers, the outer containing sodium bicarbonate and the inner containing tartaric acid. This layer was surrounded by an expansive polymeric film (composed of poly vinyl acetate [PVA] and shellac), which allowed gastric juice to pass through, and was found to swell by foam produced by the action between the gastric juices and the gas-generating agents [43]. It was shown that the swellable membrane layer played an important role in maintaining the buoyancy of the pills for an extended period of time.

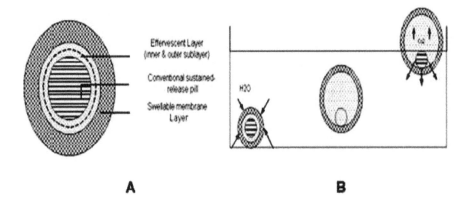

**Figure 1.6 (A) Multiple-unit oral floating drug delivery system. (B) Working principle of effervescent floating drug delivery system.**

Two parameters were evaluated: the time for the pills to be floating (TPF) and rate of pills floating at 5 hours (FP5h). It was observed that both the TPF and FP5h increased as the percentage of swellable membrane layer coated on pills having an effervescent layer increased. As the percentage of swellable layer was increased from 13% to 25% (wt/wt), the release rate was decreased and the lag time for dissolution also increased. The percentage of swellable layer was fixed at 13% wt/wt and the optimized system showed excellent floating ability in vitro (TPF ~10 minutes and FP5h ~80%) independent of pH and viscosity of the medium.

Yang et al [44] developed a swellable asymmetric triple-layer tablet with floating ability to prolong the gastric residence time of triple drug regimen (tetracycline, metronidazole, and clarithromycin) in Helicobacter pylori–associated peptic ulcers using hydroxy propyl methyl cellulose (HPMC) and poly (ethylene oxide) (PEO) as the rate-controlling polymeric membrane excipients. The design of the delivery system was based on the swellable asymmetric triple-layer tablet approach. Hydroxypropylmethylcellulose and poly (ethylene oxide) were the major rate-controlling polymeric excipients. Tetracycline and metronidazole were incorporated into the core layer of the triple-layer matrix for controlled delivery, while bismuth salt was included in one of the outer layers for instant release. The floatation was accomplished by incorporating a gas-generating layer consisting of sodium bicarbonate: calcium carbonate (1:2 ratios) along with the polymers. The in vitro results revealed that the sustained delivery of tetracycline and metronidazole over 6 to 8 hours could be achieved while the tablet remained afloat. The floating feature aided in prolonging the gastric residence time of this system to maintain high localized concentration of tetracycline and metronidazole.

Ozdemir et al [45] developed floating bilayer tablets with controlled release for furosemide. The low solubility of the drug could be enhanced by using the kneading method, preparing a solid dispersion with β cyclodextrin mixed in a 1:1 ratio. One layer contained the polymers HPMC 4000, HPMC 100, and CMC (for the control of the drug delivery) and the drug. The second layer contained the effervescent mixture of sodium bicarbonate and citric acid. The in vitro floating studies revealed that the lesser the compression force the shorter is the time of onset of floating, ie, when the tablets were compressed at 15 MPa, these could begin to float at 20 minutes whereas at a force of 32 MPa the time was prolonged to 45 minutes. Radiographic studies on 6 healthy male volunteers revealed that floating tablets were retained in stomach for 6 hours and further blood analysis studies showed that bioavailability of these tablets was 1.8 times that of the conventional tablets. On measuring the volume of urine the peak diuretic effect seen in the conventional tablets was decreased and prolonged in the case of floating dosage form.

Choi et al [46] prepared floating alginate beads using gas forming agents (calcium carbonate and sodium bicarbonate) and studied the effect of $CO_2$ generation on the physical properties, morphology, and release rates. The study revealed that the kind and amount of gas-forming agent had a profound effect on the size, floating ability, pore structure, morphology, release rate, and mechanical strength of the floating beads. It was concluded that calcium carbonate formed smaller but stronger beads than sodium bicarbonate. Calcium carbonate was shown to be a less-effective gas forming agent than sodium bicarbonate but it produced superior floating beads with enhanced control of drug release rates. In vitro floating studies revealed that the beads free of gas-forming agents sank uniformly in the media while the beads containing gas-forming agents in proportions ranging from 5:1 to 1:1 demonstrated excellent floating (100%).

Li et al [47, 48] evaluated the contribution of formulation variables on the floating properties of a gastro floating drug delivery system using a continuous floating monitoring device and statistical experimental design. The formulation was conceived using taguchi design. HPMC was used as a low-density polymer and citric acid was incorporated for gas generation. Analysis of variance (ANOVA) test on the results from these experimental designs demonstrated that the hydrophobic agent magnesium stearate could significantly improve the floating capacity of the delivery system. High-viscosity polymers had good effect on floating properties. The residual floating force values of the different grades of HPMC were in the order K4 M~ E4 M~K100 LV9 E5 LV but different polymers with same viscosity, i.e., HPMC K4M, HPMC E4M did not show any significant effect on floating property. Better floating was achieved at a higher HPMC/carbopol ratio and this result demonstrated that carbopol has a negative effect on the floating behavior.

Penners et al [49] developed an expandable tablet containing mixture of polyvinyl lactams and polyacrylates that swell rapidly in an aqueous environment and thus reside in stomach over an extended period of time. In addition to this, gas-forming agents were incorporated. As the gas formed, the density of the system was reduced and thus the system tended to float on the gastric contents.

Fassihi and Yang [50] developed a zero-order controlled release multilayer tablet composed of at least 2 barrier layers and 1 drug layer. All the layers were made of swellable, erodible polymers and the tablet was found to swell on contact with aqueous medium. As the tablet dissolved, the barrier layers eroded away to expose more of the drug. Gas evolving agent was added in either of the barrier layers, which caused the tablet to float and increased the retention of tablet in a patient's stomach.

Talwar et al [51] developed a once-daily formulation for oral administration of ciprofloxacin. The formulation was composed of 69.9% ciprofloxacin base, 0.34% sodium alginate, 1.03% xanthum gum, 13.7% sodium bicarbonate, and 12.1% cross-linked poly vinyl pyrrolidine. The viscolysing agent initially and the gel-forming polymer later formed a hydrated gel matrix that entrapped the gas, causing the tablet to float and be retained in the stomach or upper part of the small intestine (spatial control). The hydrated gel matrix created a tortuous diffusion path for the drug, resulting in sustained release of the drug (temporal delivery).

Baumgartner et al [52] developed a matrix-floating tablet incorporating a high dose of freely soluble drug. The formulation containing 54.7% of drug, HPMC K4 M, Avicel PH 101, and a gas-generating agent gave the best results. It took 30 seconds to become buoyant. In vivo experiments with fasted state beagle dogs revealed prolonged gastric residence time. On radiographic images made after 30 minutes of administration, the tablet was observed in animal's stomach and the next image taken at 1 hour showed that the tablet had altered its position and turned around. This was the evidence that the tablet did not adhere to the gastric mucosa. The MMC (phase during which large non-disintegrating particles or dosage forms are emptied from stomach to small intestine) of the gastric emptying cycle occurs approximately every 2 hours in humans and every 1 hour in dogs but the results showed that the mean gastric residence time of the tablets was 240 ± 60 minutes (n = 4) in dogs. The comparison of gastric motility and stomach emptying between humans and dogs showed no big difference and therefore it was speculated that the experimentally proven increased gastric residence time in beagle dogs could be compared with known literature for humans, where this time is less than 2 hours.

Moursy et al [53] developed sustained release floating capsules of nicardipine HCl. For floating, hydrocolloids of high viscosity grades were used and to aid in buoyancy sodium bicarbonate was added to allow evolution of $CO_2$. In vitro analysis of a commercially available 20-mg capsule of nicardipine HCl (MICARD) was performed for comparison. Results showed an increase in floating with increase in proportion of hydrocolloid. Inclusion of sodium bicarbonate increased buoyancy. The optimized sustained release floating capsule formulation was evaluated in vivo and compared with MICARD capsules using rabbits at a dose equivalent to a human dose of 40 mg. Drug duration after the administration of sustained release capsules significantly exceeded that of the MICARD capsules. In the latter case the drug was traced for 8 hours compared with 16 hours in former case.

Atyabi and coworkers [54] developed a floating system using ion exchange resin that was loaded with bicarbonate by mixing the beads with 1 M sodium bicarbonate solution. The loaded beads were then surrounded by a semipermeable membrane to avoid sudden loss of $CO_2$. Upon coming in contact with gastric contents an exchange of chloride and bicarbonate ions took place that resulted in $CO_2$ generation thereby carrying beads toward the top of gastric contents and producing a floating layer of resin beads (Figure 4). The in vivo behavior of the coated and uncoated beads was monitored using a single channel analyzing study in 12 healthy human volunteers by gamma radio scintigraphy. Studies showed that the gastric residence time was prolonged considerably (24 hours) compared with uncoated beads (1 to 3 hours).

### 1.6.2 Non-Effervescent Floating Dosage Forms

Non-effervescent floating dosage forms use a gel forming or swell able cellulose type of hydrocolloids, polysaccharides, and matrix-forming polymers like polycarbonate, polyacrylate, polymethacrylate, and polystyrene. The formulation method includes a simple approach of thoroughly mixing the drug and the gel-forming hydrocolloid. After oral administration this dosage form swells in contact with gastric fluids and attains a bulk density of < 1. The air entrapped within the swollen matrix imparts buoyancy to the dosage form. The so formed swollen gel-like structure acts as a reservoir and allows sustained release of drug through the gelatinous mass.

Thanoo et al [55] developed polycarbonate microspheres by solvent evaporation technique. Polycarbonate in dichloromethane was found to give hollow microspheres that floated on water and simulated biofluids as evidenced by scanning electron microscopy (SEM). High drug loading was achieved and drug-loaded microspheres were able to float on gastric and intestinal fluids. It was found that increasing the drug-to-polymer ratio increased both their mean particle size and release rate of drug.

Nur and Zhang [56] developed floating tablets of captopril using HPMC (4000 and 15 000 cps) and carbopol 934P. In vitro buoyancy studies revealed that tablets of 2 kg/cm2 hardness after immersion into the floating media floated immediately and tablets with hardness 4 kg/cm2 sank for 3 to 4 minutes and then came to the surface. Tablets in both cases remained floating for 24 hours. The tablet with 8 kg/cm2 hardness showed no floating capability. It was concluded that the buoyancy of the tablet is governed by both the swelling of the hydrocolloid particles on the tablet surface when it contacts the gastric fluids and the presence of internal voids in the center of the tablet (porosity). A prolonged release from these floating tablets was observed as compared with the conventional tablets and a 24-hour controlled release from the dosage form of captopril was achieved.

Bulgarelli et al [57] studied the effect of matrix composition and process conditions on casein gelatin beads prepared by emulsification extraction method. Casein by virtue of its emulsifying properties causes incorporation of air bubbles and formation of large holes in the beads that act as air reservoirs in floating systems and serve as a simple and inexpensive material used in controlled oral drug delivery systems. It was observed that the percentage of casein in matrix increases the drug loading of both low and high porous matrices, although the loading efficiency of high porous matrices is lower than that of low porous matrices.

Whitehead et al [58] prepared floating alginate beads incorporating amoxycillin. The beads were produced by drop-wise addition of alginate into calcium chloride solution, followed by removal of gel beads and freeze-drying. The beads containing the dissolved drug remained buoyant for 20 hours and high drug-loading levels were achieved.

Streubel et al [59] prepared single-unit floating tablets based on polypropylene foam powder and matrix-forming polymer. Incorporation of highly porous foam powder in matrix tablets provided density much lower than the density of the release medium. A 17% wt/wt foam powder (based on mass of tablet) was achieved in vitro for at least 8 hours. It was concluded that varying the ratios of matrix-forming polymers and the foam powder could alter the drug release patterns effectively.

El-Kamel et al [60] prepared floating microparticles of ketoprofen, by emulsion solvent diffusion technique. Four different ratios of Eudragit S 100 with Eudragit RL were used. The formulation containing 1:1 ratio of the 2 abovementioned polymers exhibited high percentage of floating particles in all the examined media as evidenced by the percentage of particles floated at different time intervals. This can be attributed to the low bulk density, high packing velocity, and high packing factor.

Illum and Ping [61] developed microspheres that released the active agent in the stomach environment over a prolonged period of time. The active agent was encased in the inner core of microspheres along with the rate-controlling membrane of a water-insoluble polymer. The outer layer was composed of bioadhesive (chitosan). The microspheres were prepared by spray drying an oil/water or water/oil emulsion of the active agent, the water-insoluble polymer, and the cationic polymer.

Streubel et al [62] developed floating microparticles composed of polypropylene foam, Eudragit S, ethyl cellulose (EC), and polymethyl metha acrylate (PMMA) and were prepared by solvent evaporation technique. High encapsulation efficiencies were observed and were independent of the theoretical drug loading. Good floating behavior was observed as more than 83% of microparticles were floating for at least 8 hours. The in vitro drug release was dependent upon the type of polymer used. At similar drug loading the release rates increased in the following order PMMA G EC G Eudragit S. This could be attributed to the different permeabilities of the drug in these polymers and the drug distribution within the system.

Javed Ali et al [39] develop a hydrodynamically balanced system of metformin as a single unit floating capsule. Various grades of low-density hydrophilic polymers were used for the formulation of this system, ,which upon contact with gastric fluid acquired and maintained a bulk density of less than 1 thereby being buoyant on the gastric contents of stomach until all the drug was released.

Kawashima et al [63] prepared multiple-unit hollow microspheres by emulsion solvent diffusion technique. Drug and acrylic polymer were dissolved in an ethanol-dichloromethane mixture, and poured into an aqueous solution of PVA with stirring to form emulsion droplets. The rate of drug release in micro balloons was controlled by changing the polymerto- drug ratio. Microballoons were floatable in vitro for 12 hours when immersed in aqueous media. Radiographical studies proved that microballoons orally administered to humans were dispersed in the upper part of stomach and retained there for 3 hours against peristaltic movements.

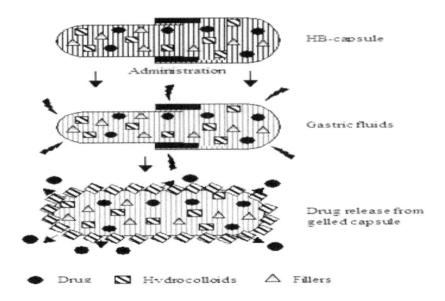

**Figure 1.6. Working principle of hydrodynamically balanced system.**

Joseph et al [64] developed a floating dosage form of piroxicam based on hollow polycarbonate microspheres. The microspheres were prepared by the solvent evaporation technique.

Encapsulation efficiency of ~95% was achieved. In vivo studies were performed in healthy male albino rabbits. Pharmacokinetic analysis was derived from plasma concentration vs time plot and revealed that the bioavailability from the piroxicam microspheres alone was 1.4 times that of the free drug and 4.8 times that of a dosage form consisting of microspheres plus the loading dose and was capable of sustained delivery of the drug over a prolonged period.

From the above discussions it is found that, the controlled gastric retention of solid dosage forms may be achieved by the mechanisms of mucoadhesion, flotation, sedimentation, expansion, modified shape systems, or by the simultaneous administration of pharmacological agents that delay gastric emptying. Among the different approaches that have been developed, low density system holds promise. Floating DDS systems are low density systems that have sufficient buoyancy to float over gastric contents, and the drug is released slowly at the desired rate, which results in increased gastro-retention and reduces fluctuations in plasma drug concentration. Both natural such as chitosan [65] and synthetic polymers (polycarbonate [55], polyacrylate [63], polymethacrylate [66, 67], polystyrene [68], ethyl cellulose [71], cellulose acetate [66, 67] etc) and some novel excipients like calcium silicate [70], low density foam powder [59] have been used to achieve floatation. One of the methods to prepare such floating microspheres is the emulsion solvent evaporation method. However literature survey revealed that very few works have been carried out so far to prepare floating microspheres of metformin HCl. Rao et al [69] designed floating microcapsules of metformin HCl using hydrophilic polymers, and concluded that HPMC has better floating ability than other hydrophilic polymers, but it cannot control the drug release for extended period of time. Ray et al [71] prepared floating controlled microcapsules of metformin HCl by emulsion solvent evaporation method using ethyl cellulose as retardant polymer. He, however reported that the prepared microcapsules have minimum floating tendency, but exhibited satisfactory drug release kinetics close to the marketed extended release tablet formulations. Therefore, it seemed reasonable to develop a gastro-retentive DDS of metformin HCl with improved buoyancy in order to optimize the pharmacokinetics and pharmacodynamics of the drug.

The author reported a simple and reproducible method for encapsulation of highly water soluble drug metformin HCl into sustained release floating microcapsules using two polymers of different permeability characteristics Cellulose Acetate Butyrate (MW of 16,000) and Eudragit RL100 (MW of 150,000), in order to achieve an extended retention in the upper GIT, which may result in enhanced absorption and thereby improved bioavailability.

## 2.1 Fundamental considerations for microencapsulation of therapeutic agents

The realization of the potential that microencapsulation offers involves a basic understanding of the general properties of microcapsules, such as the nature of the core and coating materials, the stability and release characteristics of the coated materials and the microencapsulation methods [72].

### 2.1.1 Core material

The core material, defined as the specific material to be coated, can be liquid or solid in nature. The composition of the core material can be varied as the liquid core can include dispersed and/or dissolved material. The solid core can be mixture of active constituents, stabilizers, diluents, excipients and release-rate retardants or accelerators. The ability to vary the core materials composition provides definite flexibility and utilization of this characteristic often allows effectual design and development of the desired microcapsules properties.

### 2.1.2 Coating material

The selection of appropriate coating material decides the physical and chemical properties of the resultant microcapsules/microspheres. While selecting a polymer the product requirements ie. stabilization, reduced volatility, release characteristics, environmental conditions, etc. should be taken into consideration. The polymer should be capable of forming a film that is cohesive with the core material. It should be chemically compatible, non-reactive with the core material and provide the desired coating properties such as strength, flexibility, impermeability, optical properties and stability.

Generally hydrophilic polymers, hydrophobic polymers (or) a combination of both are used for the microencapsulation process. A number of coating materials have been used successfully; examples of these include gelatin, polyvinyl alcohol, ethyl cellulose, cellulose acetate phthalate and styrene maleic anhydride. The film thickness can be varied considerably depending on the surface area of the material to be coated and other physical characteristics of the system. The microcapsules may consist of a single particle or clusters of particles. After isolation from the liquid manufacturing vehicle and drying, the material appears as a free flowing powder. The powder is suitable for formulation as compressed tablets, hard gelatin capsules, suspensions, and other dosage forms [73].

### 2.1.3 Methods for preparation of perforated floating microcapsules [66, 67]

Microcapsules containing highly water-soluble drug metformin HCl can be prepared by non-aqueous emulsion solvent evaporation method with slight modification. Microcapsules are prepared by dissolving 1:1, 1:2, 1:3 ratios of both the polymers CAB and eudragit RL100. Firstly, weighed quantity of eudragit RL100 and CAB is completely dissolved in acetone at the polymer ratio 1:1, 1:2, 1:3 but the total polymer concentration employed was 10% w/w in acetone. 5% w/w of magnesium stearate is incorporated to the above polymer mixture. Weighed quantity of metformin HCl is dispersed to the above slurry and stirred in a magnetic stirrer. The drug polymer dispersions are pressurized under $CO_2$ gas, which upon release of the pressure form cavities on the polymeric surface [67]. The porous drug polymer dispersions are then slowly introduced into 70 ml liquid paraffin previously emulsified with 1 % Span 80, while stirring at 1000 rpm held by a mechanical stirrer (Remi, Mumbai) equipped with a three-blade propeller at room temperature. The whole system is stirred for 3 hour to allow the complete evaporation of acetone. The oil layer is decanted and microcapsules are washed several times with petroleum ether (40-60°). The washed microcapsules are dried in an oven at room temperature not exceeding 25 °C.

Microcapsule containing highly water-soluble drug metformin HCl is successfully encapsulated into microcapsule using two polymers of different permeability characteristics. The above modified technique is aimed at not only to improve the buoyancy of microcapsule, but also to release the drug in the acidic pH in controlled fashion. Also, to make a formulation having density lower than the gastric contents, using mixture of two polymers of different permeability characteristics.

**Table 1: Composition of the prepared microcapsules**

| Formulation Code | Drug/Polymer ratio | Polymer concentration 10% w/w | Quantity of magnesium stearate % w/w | Stirring Speed (rpm) |
|---|---|---|---|---|
| A1 | 1:2 | RL100 | 5 | 1000 |
| B1[a] | 1:2 | CAB | 5 | 1000 |
| A1B1[a] | 1:2 | RL100,CAB (1:1) | 5 | 1000 |
| B1 | 1:2 | CAB | 5 | 1500 |
| A1B1 | 1:2 | RL100,CAB (1:1) | 5 | 1800 |

The polymers used in the fabrication of microcapsule are well established polymers for the said dosage form. The two polymers are selected in such a way that one will give initial burst release, which is essential from therapeutic point of view, while the other will control the drug release by maintaining the buoyancy. Eudragit RL100 contain higher amount of quaternary ammonium groups, which renders it more permeable. It is evident that addition of eudragit RL100 increased the permeability of the microcapsules to the surrounding dissolution medium due to the swelling nature of the polymer (Bodmeier and Chen et al [79]). In addition to this, the porous nature of the microcapsule produces an upward motion of the dosage form to float on the gastric contents. Hence, the fabricated low density system has been found to be promising over, conventional tablet formulations, as it releases the drug slowly in the stomach for gradual absorption in the intestines. The slow but complete drug release in the stomach is expected to increase bioavailability of the drug as well its complete utilization which may results to, lower dose and GI side effects.

## 3.1 Evaluation of the floating microcapsules

### 3.1.1 Yield of microcapsules

The prepared microcapsules with a size range of 251-μm were collected and weighed. The measured weight was divided by the total amount of all non-volatile components which were used for the preparation of the microcapsules [71].

% Yield = (Actual weight of product / Total weight of excipient and drug) × 100

### 3.1.2 Particle size analysis

Size distribution [74] was determined by sieving the microcapsules using a nest of standard BSS sieves (36,44,25) as well as by optical microscopy using calibrated ocular micrometer (1 ocular division= 14.26 micrometer) with stage micrometer having standard division of 10 micrometer and by counting atleast100 microcapsules. The particle size of the microcapsule prepared using 10% w/w eudragit RL100, 10% w/w CAB and combination of both the polymers at 1:1 ratio (total 10% w/w) differs significantly at the same stirring speed. When the polymer to polymer ratio was 1:1, there was formation of microcapsule with large and irregular sizes due to increase in solution viscosity of the polymers. Hence, higher agitation speed is required to prepare microcapsules of same sizes as that of single polymers alone (**Table 2**).

### 3.1.3 Viscosity of the polymer solutions

The absolute viscosity, kinematic viscosity, and the intrinsic viscosity of the polymer solutions in different solvents can be measured by a U-tube viscometer (viscometer constant at 40 0C is 0.0038 mm2/s /s) at 25 ± 0.1 °C in a thermostatic bath. The polymer solutions are allowed to stand for 24 h prior to measurement to ensure complete polymer dissolution [75].

In order to measure the relative viscosity of polymer solutions, different polymer concentrations were prepared in acetone and measured the viscosity using Ostwald viscometer.

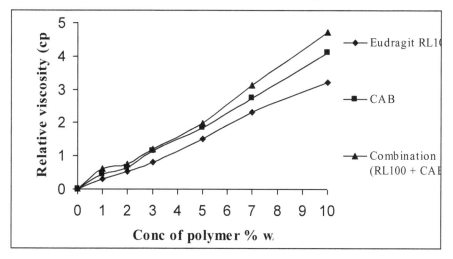

Fig 3.1.3. Relative viscosities of different concentration of eudragit RL100, CAB and combination of both the polymers at 1:1 ratio.

It is observed that CAB solutions have higher relative viscosities than those of eudragit RL100, although the later has higher molecular weight. In addition to this, solutions prepared from different concentrations of two polymers at constant 1:1 ratio have resulted in higher relative viscosities than the single polymer solution viscosities. This synergistic increase in the relative viscosity could be due to an interaction between the two polymers of different molecular weight (**Figure 3.1.3**).

### 3.1.4 Density determinations

The density of the microcapsules can be measured by using a multi volume pychnometer. Accurately weighed sample in a cup is placed into the multi volume pychnometer. Helium is introduced at a constant pressure in the chamber and allowed to expand. This expansion results in a decrease in pressure within the chamber. Two consecutive readings of reduction in pressure at different initial pressure are noted. From two pressure readings the volume and density of the microcapsule carrier is determined.

### 3.1.5 Bulk density

The microcapsules fabricated are weighed and transferred to a 10-ml glass graduated cylinder. The cylinder is tapped using an autotrap (Quantachrome, FL, USA) until the microcapsule bed volume is stabilized. The bulk density is estimated by the ratio of microcapsules weight to the final volume of the tapped microcapsules bed [76].

### 3.1.6 Angle of contact

The angle of contact is measured to determine the wetting property of a micro particulate carrier. It determines the nature of microcapsule in terms of hydrophilicity or hydrophobicity. This thermodynamic property is specific to solid and affected by the presence of the adsorbed component. The angle of contact is measured at the solid/air/water interface. The advancing and receding angle of contact are measured by placing a droplet in a circular cell mounted above objective of inverted microscope. Contact angle is measured at $20^0C$ within a minute of deposition of microcapsules [77].

### 3.1.7 Drug entrapment efficiency [66, 67]

Microcapsules equivalent to 100 mg of pure drug were crushed and added to 50 ml of 0.1M HCl, pH 1.2. The resulting mixture was shaken in a mechanical shaker for 3 hr to extract the drug completely. The solution was filtered with a Whatman filter paper and 1 ml of this solution was appropriately diluted to 25 ml using 0.1M HCl, pH 1.2, and analyzed spectophotometrically at 233 nm using Systronic 2101 UV-Visible double beam Spectro-photometer.

$$D.E.E = \frac{\text{Amount of drug actually present}}{\text{Theoretical drug load expected}} \times 100\%$$

No significant differences in drug loading for microcapsules made of different polymer solution viscosities were noted. However, the drug loading increases as the concentration of polymer is increased relative to drug concentration. The analysis of drug content showed maximum entrapment efficiency (85-90%) at the drug polymer ratio 1:2 (**Table 2**).

Table 2: Various formulation parameters for optimized floating microcapsules

| Formulation Code | Stirring speed | Particle size in micron | Drug Entrapment Efficiency (%) | Buoyancy (%) |
|---|---|---|---|---|
| A1 | 1000 | 371±3.7 | 89.35± 1.42 | 387±2.1 |
| B1[a] | 1000 | 534±1.7 | 91.51± 1.12 | 534±3.2 |
| A1B1[a] | 1000 | 710±1.4 | 90.15± 1.8 | 710±3.5 |
| B1 | 1500 | 376±1.2 | 87.31± 1.3 | 391±3.7 |
| A1B1 | 1800 | 381±0.98 | 92.07± 1.2 | 534±2.2 |

*All values are expressed as mean ± SD, n=3*

### 3.1.8 In vitro evaluation of floating ability

An in vitro floating study [29, 77] is carried out using simulated gastric fluid USP containing 0.02% Tween 80 as a dispersing medium. Microcapsules are spread over the surface of 500ml of dispersing medium at 37 ± 0.5°C. A paddle rotating at 100 rpm agitated the medium. Each fraction of microcapsules floating on the surface and those settled down are collected at a predetermined time point (upto10 hr). The collected samples are weighed after drying. The % of floating microcapsules can be determined by

$$\frac{\text{(Weight of floating microcapsules after drying)}}{\text{(Weight of floating microcapsules + settled microcapsules after drying)}} \times 100$$

Microcapsules prepared using 10% w/w CAB exhibit minimum floating ability, whereas eudragit RL100 (10% w/w) showed maximum buoyancy in 0.1M HCl. Eudragit RL100 microcapsules are found to float on gastric media for more than 10 hour. The buoyancy percentage of microcapsules prepared using combination of both the polymers at 1:1, 1:2, 1:3 ratio (total 10% w/w) are lower than that of eudragit RL100 alone. But, it is evident that, microcapsules prepared using combination of both the polymers has higher floating ability than that of CAB alone.

### 3.1.9. Scanning Electron Microscopy (SEM)

Morphology and surface topography [78] of the microcapsules are examined by Scanning Electron Microscopy (SEM, Hitachi S-3600N, Japan). The samples are mounted on the SEM sample stab, using a double sided sticking tap and coated with gold (200A°) under reduced pressure (0.001 torr) for 5 min to improve the conductivity using an Ion sputtering device. The coated samples are observed under the SEM and photomicrographs are obtained at different magnifications 20x, 40x, 200x, 400x etc.

SEM study shows that particles made of eudragit RL100 are spherical [Fig 3.1.9]. The surface of the drug-loaded microcapsules manifested the presence of drug particles, clearly visible from outside [Fig 3.1.9 (a)]. The number of pores on the microcapsules surface increases after dissolution.

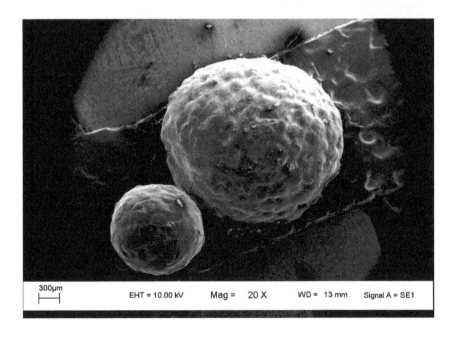

Fig. 3.1.9 (a) SEM photographs of drug loaded microcapsules made of eudragit RL100 and cellulose acetate butyrate polymers before dissolution.

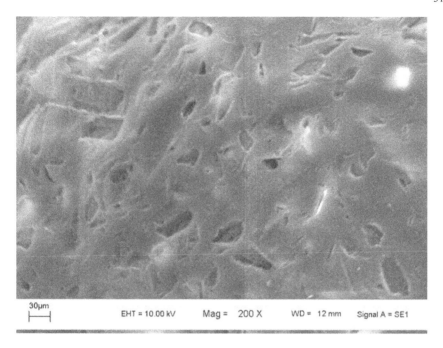

**Fig.3.1.9 (b) SEM photographs of drug loaded microcapsules made of eudragit RL100 and cellulose acetate butyrate polymers after dissolution.**

However, microcapsules made of CAB alone are smooth and spherical with no pores visible from outside and no adhering drug particles are present before dissolution [Fig 3.1.9 (a)]. SEM study clearly reveals the smoothness of the spherically shaped particles. The microcapsules prepared from the polymer to drug ratio at 2:1 has a smooth surface with many pores after the dissolution study [Fig 3.1.9 (b)]. Irregular surfaces and smaller sizes are observed in the microcapsules prepared from polymer to drug ratio 1:1. Large aggregates of magnesium stearate are visible over the microcapsules surface. Presence of pores are detected on the microcapsules surface which increased in size and number after dissolution indicating leaching of the drug through these channels. Microcapsules prepared from combination of both the polymers at different polymer to polymer ratio have more or less similar characteristics to that of CAB and eudragit RL100 microcapsules. However, the spherical nature and size of the microcapsules does not change after the dissolution tests.

## 3.1.10. Fourier Transform Infrared Spectroscopy (FT-IR)

Drug-polymer interactions are studied by FTIR spectroscopy [73]. The spectra are recorded for pure drug and drug-loaded microcapsules using FTIR (PerkinElmer, Model No. 883). Samples are prepared in KBr disks (2 mg sample in 200 mg KBr). The scanning range usually 400-4000 cm$^{-1}$ and the resolution is 2 cm$^{-1}$. While studying floating microcapsules using metformin as model drug, the principle absorption peaks of pure metformin HCl appears at 3171 cm$^{-1}$ due to the N-H stretching of the primary amine group (-NH$_2$) and at 1062 cm$^{-1}$ due to C-N stretching [Fig 3.1.10 (a)]. However, a sharp peak at 1580 cm$^{-1}$ occurs due to N-H bending vibrations of the primary amine group. There is also peaks at 2210-2260 cm$^{-1}$ due to C-N stretching of the -C=NH group. A single weak bond of 2901-3170 appears due to N-H stretching of secondary amine group.

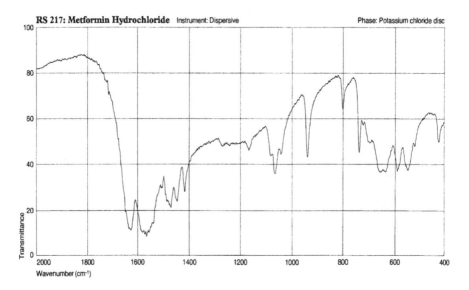

Fig 3.1.10 (a) FT-IR spectra of pure drug Metformin HCl.

The identical peaks of N-H stretching, C-N stretching, N-H bending vibrations are also appeared in the spectra of metformin loaded microcapsules prepared with eudragit RL100, CAB and Combination of both the polymers [Fig 3.1.10 (b)]. This observation indicates that no chemical interactions between the drug and the polymers used. However, slight shifts in the spectra of microcapsules are noticed as compared to the spectra of pure drug, and this may be due to the physico-chemical bonding of the drug with the polymer.

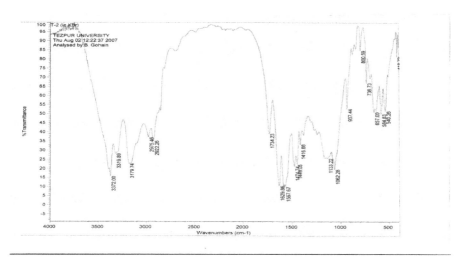

**Fig 3.1.10 (b) FT-IR spectra of drug loaded Cellulose acetate butyrate and Eudragit RL100 microcapsules.**

### 3.1.11. Differential Scanning Calorimetry (DSC)

The DSC analysis of pure drug and drug-loaded microcapsules are carried out by using a Diamond DSC (Perkin Elmer, USA) to evaluate any possible drug-polymer interaction [73]. The analysis is usually performed at a rate 5° /min from 50 ° C to 500 ° C temperature ranges under nitrogen flow of 50 ml min $^{-1}$.

DSC has been one of the most widely used calorimetric techniques to characterize the physical state of the drug in the polymer matrix. The DSC thermo gram of metformin HCl exhibited a single endothermic peak at 228.34°C corresponding to its melting transition temperature. This peak is also observed in the thermo gram of microcapsules prepared using eudragit RL100, even though slightly broadened but shifted to lower temperature at 232.50° C, which was less sharp and also a broad endothermic peak is found at 371.83° C which is due to polymer eudragit RL100. This may also be due to the fact that presence of eudragit RL100 depresses the melting point of metformin HCl and broadened its melting point endotherm. This can be further explained that presence of polymer causes a significant reduction in drug crystallinity in the polymer matrix.

### 3.1.12. X-ray powder Diffractometry [73]

X-ray powder diffractometry is carried out to investigate the effect of microencapsulation process on crystallinity of drug. Powder X-RD patterns are recorded on Seifert make Diffract meter, Japan (Model-XRD-3003 TT) using Ni-filtered, Cu k α radiation, at a voltage of 30 kV and a current of 25 mA. The scanning rate employed is 20/min, over the 4 ° to 40 ° diffraction angle (2θ) range. The X-RD patterns of drug powder and drug-loaded microcapsules are recorded.

Powder X-RD technique has been extensively utilized along with DSC to study the physical state of the drug in the polymer matrix. The crystalline nature of the metformin HCl is clearly demonstrated by its characteristics PXRD pattern containing well define peaks between 2 theta of 22 to 40 degree. There is sharp peak occurs in case of pure drug due to the diffraction of the crystalline character of the pure drug. However, The X-RD spectrum of the blank polymers eudragit RL100, CAB doesn't show any diffraction pattern due to the absence of the crystalline character, i.e. it exist in the amorphous form. However, drug loaded microcapsules prepared with the single polymers and combination polymers exhibited characteristic diffraction pattern, which is less intense as compared to pure drug. The presence of diffract gram which is much decreased in the drug loaded microcapsules indicated that drug present in the polymer matrix in crystalline state and the presence of polymer has further decreased the crystallinity of the pure drug.

### 3.1.13 Dissolution characteristics of Metformin HCl floating microcapsules

In vitro drug release studies [74] are carried out for all products in USP type II fitted with six rotating basket [Campbell Electronics, Mumbai, India] dissolution test apparatus. ). The microcapsules are evaluated for drug release using 900 ml of simulated gastric fluid (pH 1.2) and simulated intestinal fluid (pH 6.8) for 10 hour maintained at 37 ± 0.1°C and stirred at 100 rpm. 2 ml of aliquot is withdrawn at different time intervals and an equivalent volume of medium prewarmed at 37°C is added to maintain sink condition. Withdrawn samples are analyzed spectrophotometrically at 233 nm using a UV-Visible double beam Spectrophotometer (1700, Shimadzu, Japan). The concentrations of drug in test samples are corrected for sampling effect using following formula.

$$C_n = \left(\frac{Mn}{V_T - Vs}\right)\left(\frac{V_T}{M_{n-1}}\right) X\ C_{n-1}$$

Where,  $C_n$ is the corrected concentration of the $n^{th}$ sample,
$M_n$ is the original concentration of the $n^{th}$ sample,
$V_T$ is the volume of the dissolution medium,
$V_S$ is the volume of the sample withdrawn,
$C_{n-1}$ is the corrected concentration of the $(n-1)^{th}$ sample, and
$M_{n-1}$ is the original concentration of the $(n-1)^{th}$ sample

The dissolution profiles of the prepared formulations are compared with that of the marketed formulations to arrive at the target release. The selected formulations are tested for a period of 8 weeks at different storage condition of $25^0C$ and $40^0C$ with 60% RH and 75% RH, to evaluate their drug content. The percentage drug content at different temperatures after every two weeks is determined. Dissolution study of selected formulation A1B1 is carried out after subjecting the formulation for stability study. From the stability data, the formulation is found to be stable, because there is no significant change in the percentage amount of drug content. Microcapsules made of eudragit RL100 showed good flow properties, maximum floating tendency, but faster in vitro drug release rate in both simulated gastric media (pH 1.2) and phosphate buffer (pH 6.8). The prepared microcapsules showed highest drug release of 80-85% in case of D: P 1:1, [Fig 3.1.13 (a)] and 70-75% in case of D: P 1:2, [Fig 3.1.13 (c)] within 4 to 5 hours. This suggested that as the polymer concentration is increased, the

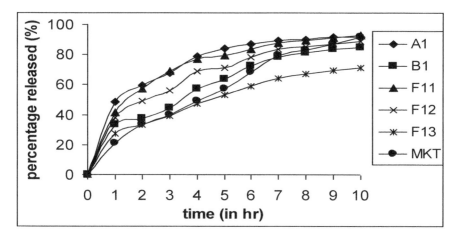

**Fig: 3.1.13 (a) Invitro drug release profiles of metformin HCl floating microcapsules in 0.1M HCl (pH 1.2) prepared using different polymer to polymer ratios (D: P 1:1) in accordance with zero order equation.**

release rate is more extended. However, all the microcapsules showed higher amount of drug release in phosphate buffer as compared to the release in 0.1M HCl.

Likewise, microcapsules made of CAB showed good flow properties, minimum floating behaviour but slower rate of invitro drug release initiated by lag time in both the dissolution media, as compared to the eudragit RL100 microspheres. It is observed from the release profile that around 50-60% in case of D: P 1:1, [Fig 3.1.13 (a)] and 40-45% in case of D: P 1:2, drug released within 4 to 5 hours [Fig: 3.1.13 (c)]. The drug release is further extended as the polymer concentration is increased. The CAB microcapsules exhibit extended release unto 10 hour, which is further extended at the drug to polymer ratio 1:2. They also showed higher amount of drug release rate in phosphate buffer as compared to 0.1M HCl.

These observations could be attributed to the fact that an increase in the polymer solution viscosity has produced microcapsules with reduced porosity due to the thickening of the polymer wall. It is understood that higher polymer concentration results in a longer diffusional path length, so drug release is extended. The thick polymeric barrier slows the entry of surrounding dissolution medium in to the microcapsules and hence less quantity of drug leaches out from the polymer matrices of the microcapsules exhibiting extended release.

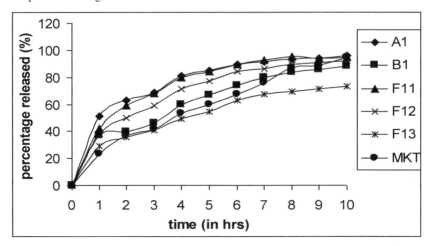

**Fig 3.1.13 (b). Invitro drug release profiles of metformin HCl floating microcapsules in Phosphate buffer (pH 6.8) prepared using different polymer-to-polymer ratios (D: P 1:1).**

### 3.1.14. Release Kinetics

In order to describe the kinetics of the release process of drugs from controlled release preparation, the data are fitted with different kinetics models [75-78]. The kinetic models used were:

(1) $Q_t = k_o\, t$  (zero-order equation)

(2) $\ln Q_t = \ln Q_0 - k_1\, t$  (first-order equation)

The first order equation describes the release from systems when dissolution rate is dependent on the concentration of the dissolving species. The Higuchi square root equation describes the release from systems where the solid drug is dispersed in an insoluble matrix and the rate of drug release is related to the rate of drug diffusion.

(3) $Q_t = K\, .S.\ \sqrt{t} = k_H\, .\ \sqrt{t}$ (Higuchi eqn based on Fickian diffusion)

Where, Q is the amount of drug release in time t, $Q_0$ is the initial amount of drug in the microcapsules., S is the surface area of the microcapsule and $k_o$, $k_1$, and $k_H$ are rate constant of zero order, first order and Higuchi rate equations respectively. In order to determine the model which will represent a best release kinetics model for the prepared formulations, the dissolution data is analyzed using the Peppas and Korsemeyer equation which is expressed as

$$M_t / M_\infty = k \cdot t^n$$

Where $M_t$ is the amount of drug release at time t and $M_\infty$ is the amount release at time $t = \infty$, thus $M_t / M_\infty$ is the fraction of drug released at time t, k is the kinetic constant, and $n$ is the diffusion exponent which can be used to characterize both mechanism for both solvent penetration and drug release.

Determining the correlation coefficient assessed fitness of the data into various kinetic models. The rate constants, for respective models were also calculated from slope. From the kinetic data it can be observed that the release of Metformin HCl from the eudragit RL100 microcapsules exhibit diffusional characteristics and highly correlated with Higuchi spherical matrix release, followed by 1st order and zero order (**Table 3**).

Table 3: Kinetic evaluation of drug release data for microcapsule formulations

| Formulation Code | Kinetic Models | | | | | | | |
|---|---|---|---|---|---|---|---|---|
| | Zero Order | | 1st Order | | Higuchi Model | | Korsemeyer Pappas Model | |
| | $R^2$ | $k_0$ | $R^2$ | $k_1$ | $R^2$ | $k_H$ | $R^2$ | n |
| A1 | 0.7531 | 6.62 | 0.9362 | 0.063 | 0.9334 | 20.49 | 0.8411 | 0.032 |
| B1 | 0.9302 | 6.02 | 0.9877 | 0.043 | 0.9721 | 22.10 | 0.9392 | 0.052 |
| A1B1 | 0.8095 | 6.26 | 0.9794 | 0.051 | 0.9741 | 20.21 | 0.8931 | 0.034 |
| MKT | 0.9671 | 8.82 | 0.9669 | 0.108 | 0.9771 | 7.51 | 0.8716 | 0.066 |

## 4.1 Conclusions

Drug absorption in the gastrointestinal tract is a highly variable procedure and prolonging gastric retention of the dosage form extends the time for drug absorption. FDDS promises to be a potential approach for gastric retention. For drugs with narrow absorption window gastroretentive controlled release floating dosage forms may produce higher bioavailability and superior effects compared to immediate release and CR oral dosage forms. This is because gradual release of the drug from the CR dosage form in the stomach results in a continuous and prolonged input of the drug to the main absorption sites located in the stomach. Although there are number of difficulties to be worked out to achieve prolonged gastric retention, a large number of research works has been carried out on the development of floating drug delivery system and are focusing toward commercializing the cost effective technique. In our study, gastric floating microcapsules of Metformin HCl was successfully prepared by using two polymers of different permeability characteristics. CAB has high butyryl content and it is insoluble at physiological pH values. CAB microcapsules extend the drug release for longer period of time, with an initial slow release at the first one hour and then controlled release for the rest period of time. But, microcapsules made of both the polymers at 1:1 ratios (total 10% w/w) exhibited satisfactory drug release pattern, as it released the drug in controlled fashion for extended period of time by maintaining the buoyancy. Although, metformin extended release tablet formulations were well established, but it causes a great fluctuations in plasma drug levels and fail to improve the bioavailability. But microcapsule formulation offer several advantages over other sustained release systems, especially matrix type tablets; since they can be widely distributed throughout the GI tract and produce local high concentration of drug at the absorption site. Therefore, it may be concluded that drug loaded floating microcapsules are a suitable delivery system for metformin with a new choice of an economical, safe and more bioavailable formulation in the management of type II diabetes mellitus.

## References

1. A .A. Deshpande, C.T. Rhodes, N.H. Shah, A.W. Malick, Controlled-release drug delivery systems for prolonged gastric residence: an overview, Drug. Dev. Ind. Pharm 1996; 22 (6):531–539.
2. B .N. Singh, K.H. Kim, Floating drug delivery systems: an approach to oral controlled drug delivery via gastric retention, J. Control. Release 2000; 63:235–259.
3. S .J. Hwang, H. Park, K. Park, Gastric retentive drug delivery systems, Crit. Rev. Ther. Drug Carrier Syst 1998; 15 (3):243–284.
4. A .J. Moes, Gastroretentive dosage forms, Crit. Rev. Ther. Drug. Carrier. Syst 1993; 10 (2):143–195.
5. Reddy LHV, Murthy RSR. Floating dosage systems in drug delivery. Crit Rev Ther Drug Carrer Syst 2002; 19(6): 553-585.
6. Talukdar R, Fassihi R. Gastroretentive delivery systems: a mini review. Drug. Dev. Ind. Pharm 2004; 30(10): 1019-1028.
7. L .H. Bannister, Alimentary system, in: P.L. Williams (Ed.) Gray's Anatomy. XXXVIII, Churchill Livingstone, New York, 1995, pp. 1683–1812.
8. T .T. Kararli, Comparison of the gastrointestinal anatomy, physiology, and biochemistry of humans and commonly used laboratory animals, Biopharm. Drug. Dispos 1995;16: 351–380.
9. W .L. Hasler, in: T.Yamada (Ed.), Textbook of Gastroenterol-ogy II, Vol. 1, J.B. Lippincott, Philadelphia, 1995, pp. 181–206.
10. J .B. Dressman, R.R. Berardi, L.C. Dermentzoglou, T.L. Russel, S.P. Schmaltz, J.L. Barnett, K.M. Jarvenpaa, Upper gastrointestinal (GI) pH in young, healthy men and women, Pharm. Res 1990; 7 (7):756–761.
11. T .L. Russell, R.R. Berardi, J.L. Barnett, L.C. Dermentzog- lou, K.M. Jarvenpaa, S.P. Schmaltz, J.B. Dressman, Upper gastrointestinal pH in seventy-nine healthy, elderly, north American men and women, Pharm. Res 1993;10 (2):187–196.

12. N .F. Barley, A. Howard, D. O'Callaghan, S. Legon, J.R.F. Walters, Epithelial calcium transporter expression in human duodenum, Am. J. Physiol. Gastrointest. Liver. Physiol 2001; 280:G285–G290.
13. S .S. Davis, E.A. Wilding, I.R. Wilding, Gastrointestinal transit of a matrix tablet formulation: comparison of canine and human data, Int. J. Pharm 1993; 94:235–238.
14. Timmermans J, Andre JM. Factors controlling the buoyancy and gastric retention capabilities of floating matrix capsules: new data for reconsidering the controversy. J. Pharm. Sci 1994; 83:18-24.
15. Wise.L.Donald.Textbook of Controlled Drug Delivery System. A Gastro retentive drug delivery system to improve oral drug delivery. Chap-24, pg.no-505-508.
16. Desai S, Bolton S. A floating controlled release drug delivery system: in vitro- in vivo evaluation. Pharm. Res 1993; 10:1321-1325.
17. S. Arora, J. Ali, A. Ahuja, R.K. Khar, S. Baboota, Floating drug delivery systems: an updated review, AAPS PharmSciTech 2005; 6:E372–E390.
18. Garg S, Sharma S. Gastroretentive drug delivery systems. Business Briefing: Pharmatech 2003; 5th edition. May 2003.
19. Ali javed, Khar RK , Ahuja alka,Sharma K.R. Formulation and development of hydro dynamically balanced system for Metformin HCl:Invitro and invivo evaluation. Eu. J.Pharm. Biopharm 2006; Dec-28.
20. Ponchel G, Irache JM. Specific and non-specific bioadhesive particulate system for oral delivery to the gastrointestinal tract. Adv. Drug. Del. Rev 1998; 34:191-219.
21. Ichikawa M, Watanabe S, Miyake Y. A new multiple unit oral floating dosage system. I: Preparation and in vitro evaluation of floating and sustained-release kinetics. J .Pharm. Sci 1991; 80:1062-1066.
22. .A. Deshpande, N.H. Shah, C.T. Rhodes, W. Malick, Development of a novel controlled-release system for gastric retention, Pharm. Res 1997; 14:815–819.
23. B. Rednick, S.J. Tucker, Sustained release bolus for animal husbandry, US patent 3 507 952, April 22 (1970).
24. R.C. Mamajek, E.S. Moyer, Drug dispensing device and method, US Patent 4, 207, 890 (1980).
25. J. Urguhart, F. Theeuwes, Drug Delivery System comprising a reservoir containing a plurality of tiny pills, US patent. 4,434,153 (1994).

26. J.A. Fix, R. Cargill, K. Engle, Controlled gastric emptying III: gastric residence time of a non-disintegrating geometric shape in human volunteers, Pharm. Res 1993; 10:1087–1089.
27. F. Fedzierewicz, P. Thouvenot, J. Lemut, A. Etinine, M. Hoffonan, P. Maincene, Evaluation of peroral silicone dosage forms in humans by gamma-scintigraphy, J. Control. Rel 1999; 58:195–205.
28. Muthuswamy K. Ravi T.K. Preparation and evaluation of lansoprazole floating micropellets. Ind. J. Pharm. Sci 2005; 67 (1):75-79.
29. Srivastava AK, Ridhurkar Rao, Waodha Saurabh. Floating microspheres of Cimetidine: Formulation, Characterization and Invitro evaluation .Acta Pharma 2005; 55:277-285.
30. Richard A. Harry, Pamela C. Champe. Lippincott's Illustrated Reviews Pharmacology, 4$^{th}$ (edn). Lippincotts Williams and Wilkins, 2009, Philadelphia.
31. Braunwald E, Fanci AS, et al (Eds): Harrison's Principles of internal medicine. 15$^{th}$ edn: Mc Graw Hill, New York, 2011.
32. (March 2010) *WHO Model List of Essential Medicines*, 16$^{th}$ edition, World Health Organization, p. 24. Retrieved on 22 December 2010.
33. Bailey CJ, Day C. Metformin: its botanical background. *Practical Diabetes International*. 2004; 21(3):115–7.
34. American Diabetes Association. Standards of medical care in diabetes—2009. *Diabetes Care*. 2009; 32 Suppl 1:S13–61.
35. Stepensky D, Friedman M, Sour W, Hoffmann A. Preclinical evaluation of pharmacokineticpharmacodynamic rationale for oral CR metformin formulation. J. Control. Release 2001; 71:107-15.
36. Marathe PH, Wen Y, Norton J et al. Wilding IR. Effect of altered gastric emptying and gastrointestinal motility on bioavailability of metformin, in: AAPS Annual Meeting, New Orleans, LA, 1999.
37. Burns SJ, Attwood D, Barnwell SG. Assesment of a dissolution vessel designed for use with floating and erodible dosage forms. Int. J. Pharm 1998; 160:213-218.
38. Joseph NJ, Laxmi S, Jayakrishnan A. A floating type oral dosage from for piroxicam based on hollow microspheres: in vitro and in vivo evaluation in rabbits. J. Control. Release 2002; 79:71-79.

39. Ali javed, Khar RK , Ahuja alka, Sharma K.R. Formulation and development of hydro dynamically balanced system for Metformin HCl:Invitro and invivo evaluation. European Journal of Pharmaceutics and Biopharmaceutics 2007; 67:196–201.
40. Yang L, Fassihi R. Zero order release kinetics from self correcting floatable configuration drug delivery system. J. Pharm. Sci. 1996;85:170-173.
41. Soppimath KS, Kulkarni AR, Rudzinski WE, Aminabhavi TM. Microspheres as floating drug delivery system to increase the gastric residence of drugs. Drug. Metab. Rev. 2001; 33:149-160.
42. Ichikawa M, Watanabe S, Miyake Y. A new multiple unit oral floating dosage system. I: Prepration and in vitro evaluation of floating and sustained-release kinetics. J. Pharm. Sci 1991; 80:1062-1066.
43. Ichikawa M, Watanabe S, Miyake Y. Granule remaining in stomach. US patent 4 844 905. July 4, 1989.
44. Yang L, Esharghi J, Fassihi R. A new intra gastric delivery system for the treatment of helicobacter pylori associated gastric ulcers: in vitro evaluation. J. Control. Release. 1999; 57:215-222.
45. Ozdemir N, Ordu S, Ozkan Y. Studies of floating dosage forms of furosemide: in vitro and in vivo evaluation of bilayer tablet formulation. Drug. Dev. Ind. Pharm 2000; 26:857-866.
46. Choi BY, Park HJ, Hwang SJ, Park JB. Preparation of alginate beads for floating drug delivery: effects of $CO_2$ gas forming agents. Int. J. Pharm 2002; 239:81-91.
47. Li S, Lin S, Daggy BP, Mirchandani HL, Chien TW. Effect of formulation variables on the floating properties of gastric floating drug delivery system. Drug. Dev. Ind. Pharm 2002; 28:783-793.
48. Li S, Lin S, Chien TW, Daggy BP, Mirchandani HL. Statistical optimization of gastric floating system for oral controlled delivery of calcium. AAPS PharmSciTech 2001; 2:E1.
49. Penners G, Lustig K, Jorg PVG. Expandable pharmaceutical forms. US patent 5 651 985. July 29, 1997.
50. Fassihi R, Yang L. Controlled release drug delivery systems. US patent 5 783 212. July 21, 1998.
51. Talwar N, Sen H, Staniforth JN. Orally administered controlled drug delivery system providing temporal and spatial control. US patent 6 261 601. July 17, 2001.

52. Baumgartner S, Kristel J, Vreer F, Vodopivec P, Zorko B. Optimisation of floating matrix tablets and evaluation of their gastric residence time. Int. J. Pharm 2000; 195:125-135.
53. Moursy NM, Afifi NN, Ghorab DM, El-Saharty Y. Formulation and evaluation of sustained release floating capsules of Nicardipine hydrochloride. Pharmazie. 2003; 58:38-43.
54. Atyabi F, Sharma HL, Mohammed HAH, Fell JT. In vivo evaluation of a novel gastro retentive formulation based on ion exchange resins. J. Control. Release. 1996; 42:105-113.
55. Thanoo BC, Sunny MC, Jayakrishnan A. Oral sustained release drug delivery systems using polycarbonate microspheres capable of floating on the gastric fluids. J Pharm Pharmacol. 1993; 45:21-24.
56. Nur AO, Zhang JS. Captopril floating and/or bioadhesive tablets: design and release kinetics. Drug. Dev. Ind. Pharm 2000; 26: 965-969.
57. Bulgarelli E, Forni F, Bernabei MT. Effect of matrix composition and process conditions on casein gelatin beads floating properties. Int. J. Pharm 2000; 198:157-165.
58. Whitehead L, Collett JH, Fell JT. Amoxycillin release from a floating dosage form based on alginates. Int. J. Pharm 2000; 210:45-49.
59. Streubel A, Siepmann J, Bodmeier R. Floating matrix tablets based on low density foam powder: effect of formulation and processing parameters on drug release. Eur. J. Pharm. Sci 2003; 18:37-45.
60. El-Kamel AH, Sokar MS, Al Gamal SS, Naggar VF. Preparation and evaluation of ketoprofen floating oral drug delivery system. Int. J. Pharm 2001; 220:13-21.
61. Illum L, Ping H. Gastroretentive controlled release microspheres for improved drug delivery. US patent 6 207 197. March 27, 2001.
62. Streubel A, Siepmann J, Bodmeier R. Floating microparticles based on low density foam powder. Int J Pharm 2002; 241:279-292.
63. Kawashima Y, Niwa T, Takeuchi H, Hino T, Ito Y. Preparation of multiple unit hollow microspheres (microballoons) with acrylic resins containing tranilast and their drug release characteristics (in vivo). J. Control. Release 1991; 16:279-290.
64. Joseph NJ, Laxmi S, Jayakrishnan A. A floating type oral dosage form for piroxicam based on hollow microspheres: in vitro and in vivo evaluation in rabbits. J. Control. Release 2002; 79:71-79.

65. El-Gibaly I. Development and in vitro evaluation of novel floating chitosan microcapsules for oral use: comparison with non-floating chitosan microspheres. Int. J. Pharm 2002; 249(1-2): 7-21.
66. Obeidat MW, Price JC. Preparation and invitro evaluation of Propylthiouracil microspheres made of CAB and eudragit RL100 by emulsion solvent evaporation method. J. Mcroencap 2005; May, 22(3):281-289.
67. Stithit S, Chen W, Price JC. Development and characterization of buoyant theophylline microspheres with near zero order release kinetics. J. Microencap 1998 Nov-Dec; 15(6): 725-37.
68. Klausner EA, Lavy E, Friedmon M et al. Expandable gastro retentive dosage forms. J. Control. Rel 2003; 90:143-162.
69. Rao V.K, Nair Subhash. Design and biopharmaceutical evaluation of gastric floating drug delivery system of Metformin HCl by using various hydrophilic polymers. Ind. J. Pharm. Edu 2006, Issue. Jan-May.
70. Jain SK, Awasthi AM, Jain NK et al. Calcium silicate based microspheres of repaglinide for gastroretentive floating drug delivery: Preparation and in vitro characterization. J .Control. Release 2005; 8:8.
71. Ray Subhabrata, Patel Asha,Thakur SR. Invitro evaluation and optimization of Controlled release Floating Drug Delivery System of Metformin HCl. DARU Pharm. 2006.Vol.14, No.2.
72. Lachman LA, Liberman HA, Kanig JL. The Theory and Practice of Industrial Pharmacy. Mumbai, India: Varghese Publishng House; 3:414-415.
73. N.K.Jain, Controlled and Novel drug delivery, 4th Edition, 236-237, 21.
74. Pao-Chu Wua, Yaw-Bin Huanga, Jui- Sheng Changa, Ming-Jun Tsaib, Yi-Hung Tsaia. Design and evaluation of sustained release microspheres of potassium chloride prepared by Eudragit. European Journal of Pharmaceutical Sciences 2003;19:115–122
75. Fang-Jing Wang, Chi-Hwa Wang. Sustained release of etanidazole from spray dried microspheres prepared by nonhalogenated solvents. J. Control. Release 2002; 81: 263–280.
76. Yi-Yan Yang, Hui-Hui Chia , Tai-Shung Chung. Effect of preparation temperature on the characteristics and release profiles of PLGA microspheres containing protein fabricated by double-emulsion solvent extraction / evaporation method. J. Control. Release 2000; 69:81–96.
77. Alagusundaram.M, Madhu Sudana chetty, C.Umashankari. Microspheres as a Novel drug delivery system – A review. International J of chem. Tech 2009: 526-534.

78. Kim Kook Chongs, Kim Mi-jung, Oh. Hee Kyong. Preparation and evaluation of sustained release microcapsules of terbutaline sulphate. Int. J. Pharm 1994, 106, pp. 213-219.
79. Bodmeier R, Chen H. Preparation and characterization of microspheres containing the anti-inflammatory agents, Indomethacin, ibuprofen and kitoprofen. J. Control. Release 1989; 10: 167-175.
80. Talukdar R, Fassinir R. Gastroretentive Delivery System: Hollow beads. Drug Dev Ind Pharm. 2004; 4:405-412.
81. Costa P, Sousa LJM. Modeling and comparision of dissolution profiles. Eu. J. Pharm. Sci 2001; 13: 123-133.
82. Costa FO, Sousa JJ, Pais AA, Fornosinho S J. Comparision of dissolution profile of ibuprofen pellets. J. Control. Release 2003; 89: 199-212.
83. Higuchi T. Mechanism of sustained action medication theoretical analysis of rate of release of solid drugs dispersed in solid matrices. J. Pharm.Sci 1963; 52: 1145-1149.
84. Peppas NA. Analysis of Fickian and non-fickian drug release from polymers. Pharm. Acta. Helv 1985; 60:110-111.

***************************

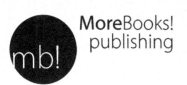
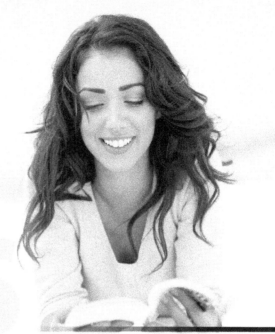

# i want morebooks!

Buy your books fast and straightforward online - at one of world's fastest growing online book stores! Free-of-charge shipping and environmentally sound due to Print-on-Demand technologies.

Buy your books online at
## www.get-morebooks.com

Kaufen Sie Ihre Bücher schnell und unkompliziert online – auf einer der am schnellsten wachsenden Buchhandelsplattformen weltweit! Versandkostenfrei und dank Print-On-Demand umwelt- und ressourcenschonend produziert.

Bücher schneller online kaufen
## www.morebooks.de

 VDM Verlagsservicegesellschaft mbH
Dudweiler Landstr. 99  Telefon: +49 681 3720 174   info@vdm-vsg.de
D - 66123 Saarbrücken  Telefax: +49 681 3720 1749  www.vdm-vsg.de

www.ingramcontent.com/pod-product-compliance
Lightning Source LLC
Chambersburg PA
CBHW062209270225
22719CB00007B/101